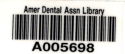

DATE DUE

```
D88 M388 2003          75089
Massotto, Mike.
The 25 sure fire ways to
  destroy your dental ...
```

Department of Library Services
American Dental Association

211 East Chicago Avenue
Chicago, Illinois 60611

REGULATIONS FOR CIRCULATION OF BOOKS

Books may be retained by members of the Association for four weeks after receipt. If they are not reserved for someone else the time will be extended on request. Borrowers are expected to replace or pay for books which are lost or damaged while in circulation. Your cooperation in returning books promptly will be **appreciated.**

GAYLORD FG

Dedication

This book is dedicated to the one doctor who truly epitomizes all 25 of the chapters in this book. May he someday see the light.

Copyright ©2003 Mike Massotto and Gary Kadi

All rights reserved. No part of this publication may be reproduced, stored in a retrieval system or transmitted in any form or by any means electronic, mechanical, photocopying, recording or otherwise, without the prior written permission of the publisher.

Published by
RJ Communications LLC
51 East 42nd Street,
Suite 1202, New York, NY 10017

Design and layout
Donna Visco

Printer
Bang Printing
3323 Oak Street, Brainerd, MN 56401

International Standard Book Number (ISBN)
Hard cover: 0-9741237-0-6

Printed in the United States of America

The 25 Sure Fire Ways To Destroy Your Dental Practice

by

Mike Massotto

and

Gary Kadi

Acknowledgements

This book is an expression of our often bizarre and crazy journey in the field of dental consulting and practice management. Our sincere gratitude and many thanks go out to all of our past and present clients who have inspired us to write this book. Thank you for providing us countless stellar examples of how to destroy a dental practice. Without you, we could not possibly have thought this stuff up.

To our world-class assistants, Jacquie and Lila, who daily do the work of ten people. Your expertise, caring, and professionalism have allowed us to grow both as a company as people. Without you, we could never serve our clients with such impeccability. To Donna Visco, whose caring and talent graces every page of this book.

Thank you,
Mike and Gary

To my wife Nancy, whose love defines the expression "soul mate", and who gives selflessly of herself in supporting all that I do. Thank you for your unconditional love despite all of the challenges that I constantly put before you with the often blind expectation of your patience and understanding. I can think of no other person in this world who I'd rather be on this adventure with.

To my son Michael, who has taught me the true meaning of love and responsibility. Hopefully someday you will read this book and not disown your father.

To my family who has yet to disown me even though in their minds I have given them numerous reasons to do so. Thank you for loving the black sheep as much as you love the others.

Finally to my mentors and coaches, past and present, who have given generously of their time, wisdom and expertise so that I could become more able and talented as a person and a coach; Ray Marquardt and Dr. David Singer who saw the diamond in the rough; and to my pop-pop Cangialosi, who I listened to when often no one else did, thank you for teaching me that life is an adventure and that it's okay to be a rebel and still be loved.

Thank you all,
Mike

To my best friend and lover, my wife, Judith. Thank you from the bottom of my heart for all the care and support you generously give every day- with you I believe anything and everything is always possible. Thank you for the many gifts you give me!

To my mentors and coaches, past and present, who have challenged me to attain new levels of personal and professional growth; my grandfather, Nicholas Abruzzi, my uncle Mike Abruzzi; Rodger Lane, Ray Marquardt, and Alice Duquesne.

To my loving family; my mom, Marie, my dad Ron; my sis Barb and her husband Mark; my grandpops, who for the past 39 years, has provided me the foundation and security to take chances everyday without fail; thank you for your wisdom, love, and support in having me achieve the amazing life that I have today.

To my dear loyal friends; Anthony, Carmello and Greg for your support, and for providing a constant reminder about the importance of having a well-balanced, fun and fulfilled life.

Thank you all,
Gary

Introduction

Why Learning How to Destroy Your Dental Practice Is Important

After years of dental consulting, we have come to discover 25 no-fail ways to ruin a dental practice. Our discoveries are based on real practices and actual experiences. During our work, we have found that it is very easy to lose sight of all the creative ways you can subconsciously, unconsciously and otherwise unwittingly do yourself in with the climate of personal and business improvement that we live in today. It is also just as easy to overlook all of the nice intentionally harmful and destructive actions you may be involved in and perhaps fail to recognize their effectiveness in facilitating your demise. Obviously there aren't many books and consulting programs on how to wreck your practice. For these reasons, we have written this book. Consider it a primer on the fundamentals of practice sabotage.

Be warned, however, for if it is not your intention to destroy your practice, and with it the rest of your life and the lives of many others near and dear to you, we suggest you read no further. For the particularly bright and ingenious, this book offers a virtual blueprint for success – in reverse. Trace the route to upset, despair, loss, financial ruin, and loneliness…then go in exactly the opposite direction and you can wind up with prosperity, happiness and fulfillment-the likes of which you may have never thought possible. Why you would want to do this is beyond us, but if you insist, be our guest.

In any event, let the advice put forth in this book speak for itself. If you don't find it at all compelling or interesting, there is truly no hope for you. You are far too ethical, sane, and success-minded to embrace the brilliance that graces these pages. However, if havoc and ruin are what you're up to, the wisdom contained herein is just what the doctor ordered.

If, by the time you've reached the end of this book, you find that you already knew all the ways to destroy your practice, then you never needed our guidance and enlightenment in the first place. You were just born with the natural ability to fail and create misery around you.

So, follow these 25 rules to the letter and you're guaranteed disaster. Avoid them and you're assured success!

Contents

Acknowledgements . . . . *II*
Introduction . . . . *V*

The 25 Sure Fire Ways To Destroy Your Dental Practice

1. Realize That It is Not a Business That You Are Running 3
2. Treat Your People Like Dirt 7
3. Nickel and Dime People to Death 11
4. Overcharge as Often as You Can Get Away With 15
5. Hire Fast, Fire Fast 19
6. Be Offensive 23
7. Resist Change 25
8. Keep Your Personal Life in a Shambles (and Bring Your Troubles To the Office) 29
9. Don't Educate Your Patients 33
10. Be as Serious as Possible 37
11. Hate Kids 41

12. Make it a Dead-End Job
   for Everyone Except You 43
13. Insist on Being Right z
   about Everything all the Time 47
14. Trust No One 51
15. Pump All of Your Money into Marketing 55
16. Never Be on Time 59
17. Don't Keep Your Word about Anything 63
18. Create a Chaotic Work Environment 67
19. Work First, Family Second 71
20. Hire a Slave, not an Associate 75
21. Keep a Lawyer in Your Back Pocket 79
22. Keep Your Facility Like a Pig Sty 83
23. Make a Lot of Enemies 87
24. Cut Corners 90
25. Start the Day with a Large Dose
   of Anti-Depressants 95

Afterward *98*

"You know the universe provides and dental school taught you plenty about running a successful practice anyway, so why sweat it?"

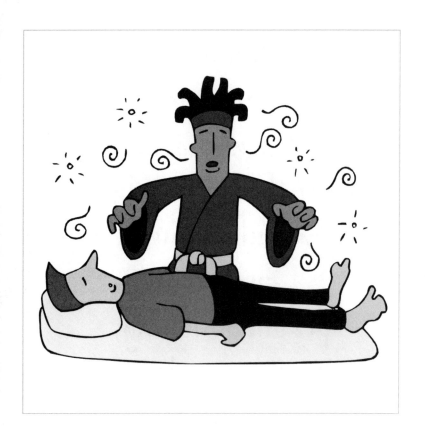

1

Realize That It is Not a Business That You Are Running

Your practice is a public sanctuary for healing. A sort of Mother Teresa meets Albert Schweitzer-type place where you fight the good fight and perform God's work as a missionary in the fight against poor dental health. So, what's business got to do with it? That's right, absolutely nothing!

Why waste valuable time that you could be spending on performing miracles of the mouth on such ridiculous frivolity as accounting, bookkeeping, paying taxes, balancing a budget, ordering supplies, training and managing staff, systematizing, implementing policy, keeping statistics, having staff meetings, and so on? All of this is the crap of corporate America which should not concern you in the least since you are a healer, not a business person. The *last* thing a healer needs is a lot of entrepreneurial hoo-hah jamming up his energy field.

You know the universe provides and dental school taught you plenty about running a successful practice anyway, so why sweat it? Business matters just have a way of taking care of themselves, as demonstrated in your practice countless times a day. Lab work not in yet? No problem, it will be there soon enough. Front desk called out sick? Hey, there's always someone around that can cover it. Patient owes for his 14 crowns, six veneers, and a bridge? Just shoot them out a kind letter and they will get right on it and pay before you know it. Hygiene schedule a little light? Isn't there a basement you've been meaning to have cleaned out or something else productive to do? So, why worry?

Anyway, none of this really matters because you have a secret ally in your corner. A behind-the-scenes entity that's always making sure the money is rolling in and you don't go broke – insurance companies (in particular HMO's). When all else fails in business, your financial future is in good hands. So leave the business management baloney to the economics majors and those high-priced practice management consultants so you can stick to healing the sick and building up more of that good karma.

"People are unimportant, and are certainly less important than you."

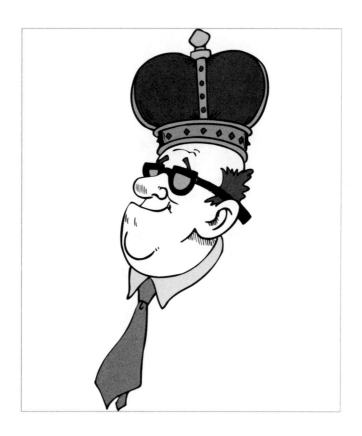

2

Treat Your People Like Dirt

In case you have not caught on yet, your staff loves to be treated like the low-life peons that they are. Be disrespectful. Be unappreciative. Never compliment or reward your staff. Treat everyone as inferior. After all, you're the one with all the fancy degrees and accolades (you have the plaques on the wall to prove it). What the hell have they ever accomplished? Most of them are boring, uneducated housewives out of retirement or working moms that probably shouldn't have gotten knocked up in the first place. They are truly lucky that you condescended and gave into their groveling to allow them to work in your palace of a practice. They barely deserve the minimum wage the government forces you to pay them, let alone the annual review and incentive plan they have been requesting. How dare they expect to make a living off of your practice? What did they invest in it to get it off the ground? You assumed all of the risk and now you and only you are due the fruits of your efforts. You are the king. That's right, king. King Cavity, King Crown, or whatever you want to call yourself. Ralph Kramden had it right 50 years ago and it still rings true today.

Acknowledgement for a job well done? Appreciation for that extra effort and overtime put in? Nonsense. These are the traits of your weak, airy-fairy competitors who don't know a damn thing about inspiring and motivating their people. You rule with an iron hand, and if anybody steps out of line (like requesting a day off for their grandmother's funeral or having to come in late after rushing their sick brat to the hospital with an appendicitis), always be sure to threaten them by holding their job in constant jeopardy. There are plenty of good laborers out there who you can snap up in a heartbeat who are better trained, will work for less money, and won't annoy you with the nuisance of having relatives die all the time, screwing up your production.

People are unimportant, and are certainly less important than you are. Besides, you're the one with the sign out front. So give them as little attention and regard as possible, berate them loudly and often (especially in front of others), and they will continue to produce for you because you pay them and give them the privilege of working for you.

"Never—I mean never—order in lunch for your people or have birthday parties, holiday parties, or any other celebration that will tap into your cash flow."

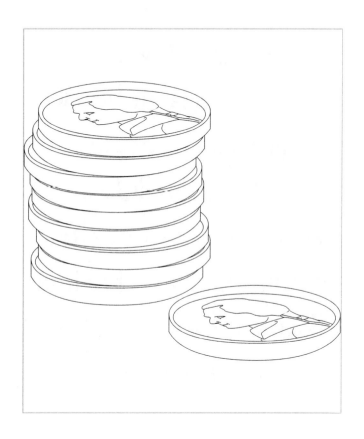

3

Nickel and Dime People to Death

If you are already treating your people like dirt, this one should be easy and a natural progression on the road to destroying your practice. Just so you know, people, particularly your staff and patients, are out to rob you blind. They want their just desserts and they see a cash cow in you. Every day they see your fancy 700 series BMW (parked in the "King Dentist-Reserved" space, of course.) That damn bookkeeper of yours has let the entire staff know just how much you're pulling in each month. They know you didn't get that new Rolex for a graduation present. So the key is to stay one step ahead of them.

Charge for every little thing and never pay for anything ever and you'll be on your way to hoarding all the extra money you'll need to keep the circling wolves at bay. Those high fear patients giving you trouble? Immediately up the bill for tolerance. Someone's hygiene visit went over by two minutes? Send a bill for the difference. Staff scrubs looking a little shabby? Be sure the new ones come out of their next paycheck. You made an extra million this year? Tell your people "Sorry, but the bonus kicks in at an extra one point five. You get the idea. Oh, and be sure to make up for the 40% discount you give for staff and family dentistry by raising your regular fees by an additional 40% for this type of work beforehand. That should even things out quite nicely. If they can't afford it, you can always give them the courtesy of docking their paycheck for the next several weeks or years if thats what it takes because that's just the kind of thoughtful leader you are.

Another tip is to make sure you never have your wallet with you at staff functions like dinners and seminars. However, should you forget to forget, be sure that everyone pays their full share including their part of the gratuity. Never-I mean never-order in lunch for your people or have birthday parties, holiday parties, or any other celebration that will tap into your cash flow. The cheaper the better is your motto. Equipment, materials, and especially people need to be gotten on the cheap. Always hire from unemployment agencies and junior high school continuing education programs. If those don't work for you, illegal aliens and ex-cons are both acceptable alternatives, which will provide you with years of quality, reliable service at a low rate of pay.

"Your patients don't know their asses from their elbows when it comes to dentistry, so you can get away with just about anything if it sounds good."

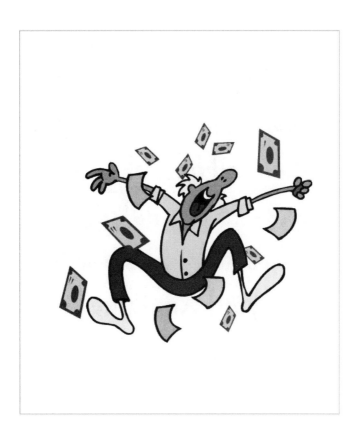

4

Overcharge as Often as You Can Get Away With

You know those late night T.V. commercials with the 1-800-DRFRAUD number that flashes across the screen as some pathetic loser of a doctor sits at his desk with his hands cupped over his face in anguish and disgrace because he finally got snagged for being an unethical thief from an anonymous tip from one of his patients? That's never going to happen to you because you are way smarter than that guy.

First of all, you have the two biggies going in your favor. Number one, your patients aren't the low-life dirt-bags like the doctor's in the commercial, and number two, they are all oblivious, friggin, morons! Your patients don't know their asses from their elbows when it comes to dentistry, so you can get away with just about anything if it sounds good. For example: "Ah, Ms. Smith, I am sorry to inform you that you are going to need 32 crowns." "But doctor, don't I have only 28 teeth left in my mouth?" "Trust me Ms. Smith, four of them are in pretty bad shape, and besides, who's the doctor here?" You get the idea – clueless. Double-decker veneers (inside and out for your viewing pleasure), Invisalign those crooked baby teeth, Nite-White one-year treatment plans...the possibilities are endless. Should you get a real sucker in your chair, try expanding your scope of practice to make a few extra bucks (i.e., "Yes Ms. Smith the cavitron will do wonders for your bunions"). Oh and by the way, didn't God give people five tooth surfaces for a reason? Not quite a root canal? Just get down to the nerve pulp and move the process along a little. Trust me, the patient will thank you for it later.

Your assistants, hygienists, and treatment coordinators are completely in the dark when it comes to this sort of thing as well. They will all mindlessly serve their master regardless of what you do because after all they don't know anything anyway and they are loyal to the end, filled with warm fuzzy feelings from all of your daily lying, cheating and stealing that they are witness to and turn the other cheek for the good of you and the practice.

"Doing due diligence on people is for attorneys and private investigators, and this is not brain surgery, astrophysics, or rocket science after all — it's dentistry."

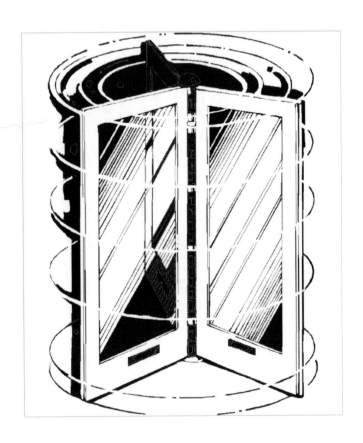

5

Hire Fast, Fire Fast

Here's a great team morale booster and another quick and easy way to put your practice into the crapper. Hire new staff as quickly as you can and throw them to the wolves – they'll be just fine. After all, you have a happy, dedicated hard-working team of helpful individuals who can't wait to take in your next victim on the hit parade and make them feel right at home. They don't mind in the least where they came from, how they got there, or just how mentally unbalanced your new hires are because it just adds to the office intrigue and makes the day that much more exciting. We can't have the practice getting boring now, can we?

Doing due diligence on people is for attorneys and private investigators, and this is not brain surgery, astrophysics, or rocket science after all – it's dentistry. It's a close-knit, transient community where people like to hop from practice to practice time and time again. So don't let those 12-page resumes concern you. Even if you have heard something negative about the person you want to bring on board (be it stealing, disruptive behavior, missed work time, poor people skills, etc.), disregard it. After all, the dentists she worked for prior to you were a big bunch of idiots who couldn't manage people to save their souls and probably got what they deserved. The new hire will be just fine with you because you're different and your practice is a much better place to work than those other dumps.

Please be sure to dismiss with the time consuming inconvenience of working interviews, employment agreements, training, and apprenticeships because it's all a waste of precious time – these new people have work to do, don't they? Time is money and it costs you valuable production time to have new people standing around observing everything all over again…Aren't these people dental professionals with years of experience under their belts? And besides, you're able to spot a good person just like that, and your flawless judgment in understanding human nature hasn't failed you yet.

Remember that nothing lasts forever anyway, so you can always fire these new people as quickly as you got them in. Who cares? They can collect unemployment, you can easily invest the equivalent of another six months of their salary in the recruiting and hiring process for their replacement, and your staff didn't get too attached to them in the first place. So, no harm done.

Actually to wrap this one up, here's a bonus little secret that works even better. Instead of firing fast, fire slow. That's right, keep the bad apples around. No need to be hasty because you want to make damn sure that these people aren't the best fit for your practice before you lose face with the rest of the staff by admitting a mistake in hiring them in the first place. Besides you can't allow any "holes in the infield" so to speak and you need bodies to run the place successfully. Take your time, get all of your ducks in a row, and if they don't flinch after several months of playing chicken, then, and only then, pull the plug.

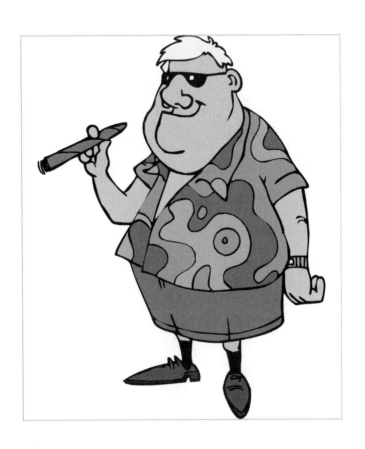

6

Be Offensive

Contrary to popular belief, dentists should smell. Bad body odor, bad breath, and liberal amounts of fragrant cologne or after-shave are the keys to success. With that handled, long, dirty fingernails (or chewed down to the cuticles instead) and tuffs of ear and nose hair make for additional professional presentation. And who said cleanliness is next to godliness has anything to do with dentistry? The place is already sterile enough, don't you think?

Matted, greasy, unkempt hair, and unstylish soiled clothing or scrubs, particularly stained with blood, sweat, and glove powder are true marks of just how hard you work. They also give the operatory that nice M*A*S*H* 4077th feel especially if you can get your hands on some Hawaiian shirts and beach sandals or clogs to complete the look.

Smoke a lot around the office (but not too close to the oxygen), because reeking of cigarettes, cigars, pipe tobacco, or better yet, the ganja, lets your patients and staff know that you have a social life and like to party. So add a few drinks to the lunch tab prior to the afternoon shift and you'll be styling.

Use of foul language is perfectly acceptable because it accentuates just how strongly you feel about others and their petty foibles, or in the case of your staff, their raging incompetence. So let it rip. And while we're on the subject, better to let loose with a good belch or expression of flatulence than risk the discomfort. Remember: it's dental hygiene that rakes in the dough, not personal hygiene.

Now for the piece de resistance – have bad teeth. Make sure you provide a stellar example of how exactly not to have your teeth look so your patients will do the opposite and pursue a healthy, good looking smile. Your patients will always do as you say-not as you do.

7

Resist Change

"Out with the old, in with the new" is definitely not your motto. Nothing could be better for the ongoing improvement and transformation of your practice than healthy, productive, well-managed and executed change – so it is to be avoided like the plague. Everyone knows that people hate change, so why deal with all the resistance? Intraoral cameras, digital x-rays, computerized files and appointment books, and while you're at it, nitrous oxide, are just plain senseless wastes of money. Sure, these luxuries are designed for the ease, comfort, and service of your staff and patients, but they don't deserve them-they already have it too damn good in life. All these people do is take, take, take, and want more, more, more as a result. Remember when you stopped using ether and leeches? That's right, everyone was so overjoyed they kept pushing for more. If you didn't stop the sudden rash of change that overcame you, the next thing you know everyone would have been pushing you to get a practice management consultant or to use lead vests when taking x-rays – and you know how expensive that type of stuff can be.

Quite frankly, change in practice is the sure route to insanity. How are you supposed to get into a nice, comfortable rut for your slow descent into early retirement (or early suicide if you prefer)? Sure as hell not with all that change going on. So don't change a thing if you know what's good for you. If it's not cancer, the IRS, or Bin Laden, why worry?

"To really speed up the practice destruction process, be sure to air all of your dirty laundry to your patients and staff."

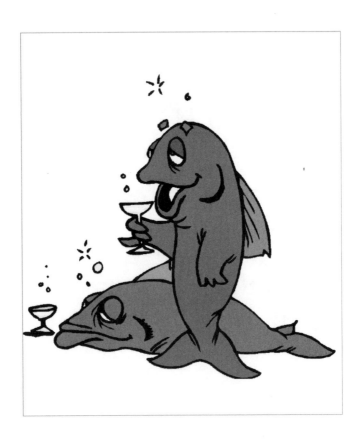

8

Keep Your Personal Life in a Shambles
(and Bring Your Troubles to the Office)

Cheat on your spouse. Beat your children. Drink like a fish. Get high as a kite. Gamble and spend like a drunken sailor. Hire prostitutes. Steal from your associates. Have an intense interest in pornography. Misuse firearms. Be in an abusive, unloving relationship. Rack up a ton of debt. Don't pay your bills. That should cover it.

    To really speed up the practice destruction process, be sure to air all of your dirty laundry to your patients and staff. Regale them with your lusty tales of marital infidelity and raucous drunken binges. Top the day off with a few dirty jokes and some sexual innuendo for the ladies in particular (see chapter six on "Being Offensive"). Hey, and doesn't sleep dentistry have its hidden advantages (wink, wink)?

Your creditors are a big bunch of bastards, aren't they? So why pay them? Make them sweat it out and wait just like your patients. You pay your debt to society everyday just by showing up at your office, you miracle worker you. If anything, they owe *you* for allowing them the honor of being on your collections list. The IRS? Don't even go there. You know that federal income tax is unconstitutional, and since you're a card carrying member of the NRA (with a human-shaped target cut out on your office door to prove it), you always have good ole' Chuck Heston to fall back on.

But all of this is quite inconsequential because of the fascinating drama that constantly surrounds and permeates your life. People find you so entertaining or feel so sorry for you they just give you a pass, rationalizing it all away. You sure don't want to be pegged as some kind of holy roller. So save the ethics and morality for Sunday, and put your attention on the most important thing in life – the moolah!

"Patients come to your office with their fears, concerns, and dental health objectives, already telepathically relayed to you and your staff, so all you have to do is dive right in and treat."

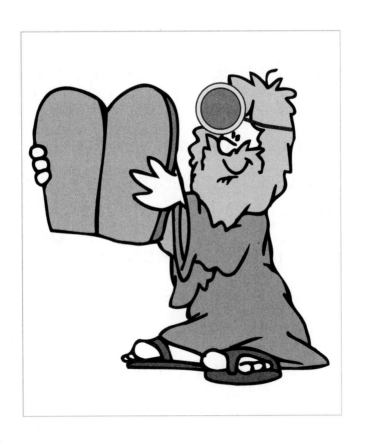

9

Don't Educate Your Patients

If there's one thing you need to know about people coming in to your dental practice, it's that they are dumber than stumps. That's right, complete ignoramuses who are there simply to piss you off and test your patience – not to mention your god-like intelligence. These people are as confused as baby raccoons. They wouldn't know a composite from an amalgam if it bit them on their derrieres, which is what most of them think with in the first place.

Face it. You're never going to get anywhere in practice bogged down chair side with models, charts, viewboxes, and taking pretty mouth pictures to wow and amaze these aghast dimwits who didn't have the common sense to peruse a few textbooks or dental journals prior to showing up in your office. The nerve of it all is not only do they expect you to fix their teeth, they want the Cliff Notes version of dental school in five minutes flat! When the Romans coined the word "doctor" for teacher they were referring to the phd's not you. But you already knew that, didn't you?

What these people have to learn how to do is just shut up, lie there, and believe every word that comes out of your mouth as if you were Moses dictating from the Mount. All you need is a little faux Burning Bush in the corner of your operatory and you're good to go. If after all of your orating they still seem a bit perplexed, remind them that you endured seven years of higher education, an internship, and a residency just so you'd have all the answers and save them the trouble.

Your word is law. Trust, rapport, and understanding have no place in the dental field. Patients come to your office with their fears, concerns, and dental health objectives already telepathically relayed to you and your staff, so all you have to do is dive right in and treat. One final note, should a patient's mouth not look bad or feel bad, not to worry. He knows that you have his best interest at heart. So start drilling and filling because an ounce of prevention is worth a pound of cure in your patient's mind.

"So serious up fast and show everyone that you're just as miserable as they are."

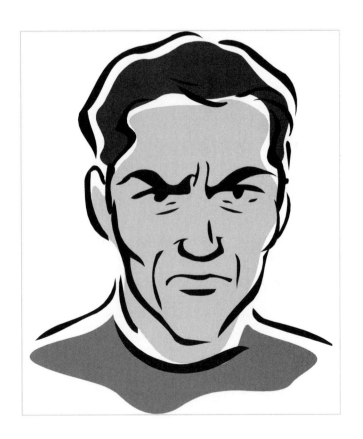

10

Be as Serious as Possible

Here's the secret to having everything go right in practice: seriousness. That's right, the more you can effort it all, the better. Put your nose to the grindstone. Work 12 hour days, six days a week (with a half day on Sunday, of course). Run the place like Mussolini and the world will be your oyster, my friend. The more solid and serious you can get, the better you will do. How solid and serious you may ask? Imagine yourself as a slab of Formica and that your work consists of joyless, unfulfilling, pseudo-medical, thankless toil. There's no time for fun and games. No one can tell if you're smiling behind your mask all day so why bother? Give it up. Medical doctors don't need all that fluffy, feel-good, lovey-dovey stuff and they do just fine. How's it gonna look if you're happy go lucky when everybody around you is upset or in pain from all the discord you cause? They ain't buyin' it, that's for sure. So serious up fast and show everyone that you're just as miserable as they are.

Now that you know that work and play have nothing to do with one another, you need to handle the epidemic of goodwill and family environment being generated by your staff before it gets completely out of hand and you start getting referrals. The last thing you need is your people slacking off with all this mirth and merriment going on. Look, if they want to feel good about themselves and their lives, send them all home early to watch, "It's a Wonderful Life" four or five times, off the clock. That should flush it out of their systems and get them back to their serious ways of pounding out the production.

"Besides, you've seen enough historical examples to know by now that kids are mischievous, malicious, loud, ill-mannered and they bite!"

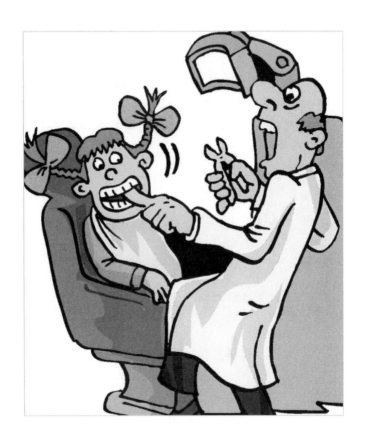

11

Hate Kids

Oh those annoying little urchins…Every time they show up in your office the entire day comes to a grinding halt. First the appointment desk, then your treatment coordinator, next your assistants, and before you know it, it's like a big friggin' Cub Scout bake-sale right in your waiting room. All the hugging and kissing and oohing and aahing, while the only thing you want is for these squirming little brats to be sitting still, aahing and oohing as you jab them full of Novocain in your dental chair. Of course while the entire staff is involved in this pseudo - PTA slack fest, where's little Johnny or Suzy? Off busting something valuable, that's where! Remember that beautiful aquarium you used to have filled with thousands of dollars of tropical fish that's now a terrarium? Besides, you've seen enough historical examples to know by now that kids are mischievous, malicious, loud, ill-mannered and they bite! Therefore, they have no place in your office.

As a matter of fact, kids should be illegal and

banned - rounded up by sadistic, dog catcher-like, goblins with mobile cages disguised as ice cream trucks and locked away in a dungeon at least until they're 10, and old enough to need root canal. Hey, it worked in that timeless classic Chitty Chitty Bang Bang, and it can work for you too. Until they pass legislation supporting this, however, you best save yourself the trouble, and pawn the pee-wees off on the associate. If you want them out of your office for good, just skip numbing them up. It works like a charm and, before you know it, your practice will be free and clear of kids who, as you know, grow-up and neglect paying you just like their thieving parents.

In short, kids are the bane of your practice. Disdain them, avoid them, and at best, have no patience for them until they are adults. By then they will have forgotten all about their early dental experiences and come running back to you with outstretched arms for all their dental needs.

12

Make it a Dead-End Job for Everyone Except You

Look, the bottom line is, you're going places and you can't afford to let anyone get in your way – particularly your staff and associates. The sooner you realize these people are nothing more than parasitic drones that are going no where fast, the sooner you will be rolling in dough at the top of your profession, baby. Sure, you probably have treating your people like dirt while nickel and diming them to death down to a science, and you have hired a mindless automaton for an associate, haven't you? All well and good, but you need to make it painfully apparent to these thralls early on that they should get any crazy ideas about raises, promotions, and partnerships out of their minds in a hurry. If you don't, you'll soon find yourself surrounded by self-motivated, entrepreneurial thinkers demanding practice improvement and expansion all at your expense! What's worse, is you'd be forced to give up absolute dictatorial control over everything in your practice and you know what happens then, don't you? Correct again, Dr. Napoleon – total anarchy. Now you can see how vital it is to keep down the masses because if you don't you may find yourself exiled to an island off the coast of Italy along with the thousands of other dentists who were too slow or too stupid to realize that giving away some power was the beginning of their demise in practice. Luckily for you, you picked up this book and are committing it to memory.

As a last bit of advice be very careful never to invest a cent in the training or development of your people. Seminars, workshops, boot camps, and personal coaching are for your eyes and ears only. The amount of money you spend on this type of stuff for your people is inversely proportional to the degree of back-stabbing and mutiny you risk suffering. So, Dr. Bligh, run the practice like the *Bounty* and reap the spoils of your success which you and only you so richly deserve.

"The annoying thing about human nature as it relates to your practice is that people like to be right — your staff, your patients, your associates and yes, even your spouse feel it constantly necessary to be right about everything, and yet they never are."

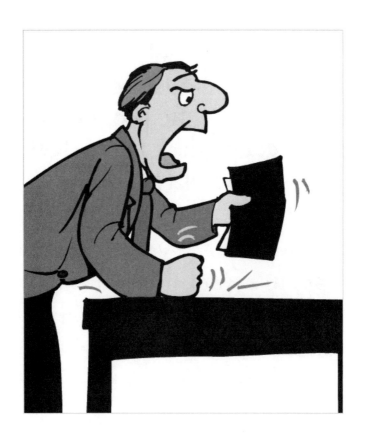

13

Insist on Being Right about Everything all the Time

It's a well-known fact that you are never wrong. The problem is, everyone else has not caught on to this yet—as unfathomable as it may seem. The annoying thing about human nature as it relates to your practice is that people like to be right – your staff, your patients, your associates and yes, even your spouse, feel it constantly necessary to be right about everything, and yet they never are. Only you have been bestowed this gift of god-like omniscience far superior to the mere mortals who have not even spent a day in your shoes. How could they possibly know what you know or have the unmitigated gall to suggest they may know something you don't? Their advice is flawed, their counsel shoddy, and their ideas, if they haven't been stolen from you, are pathetically flimsy to say the least. Look, you didn't get as far as you've gotten in practice and in life being wrong, have you? People out to make you wrong don't know who they're messing with. You'll stand for none of it. Your dentistry is 100% flawless and masterful every time unless, of course, your hygienist, assistant, the lab, or the patient himself wrecks it in some way. Your conduct is consistently appropriate and professional in every way-in and out of the office. Your superior business sense and people empathy put you on a separate plane of existence. So only rightness and goodness flow from you, you angel of mercy you. To err is human and to forgive divine, and brother don't you earn your wings every day with all the mistakes, gaffs, and blunders you endure. If everyone would just defer to you, you wouldn't have to waste so much time and effort blaming, demeaning, and correcting others all day long.

A final note on being right is to make sure you're asserting the fact that you are right all the time. It's never enough to be content with knowing you are right and the other person is wrong. You must be sure to prove it to them and everyone else in your sphere of influence so there is no doubt who the supra-genius is in these parts.

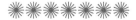

"Don't take risks, be leery of people's intentions, and when in doubt know they are trying to take advantage of you."

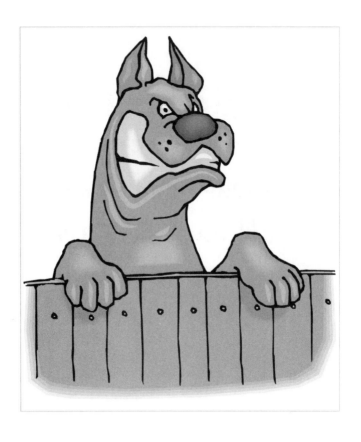

14

Trust No One

Don't take risks, be leery of people's intentions, and when in doubt, know they are trying to take advantage of you. Give your staff an inch and expect they'll take a mile. Cut a patient a break, and you can be sure they'll expect the same every time they come in. Be safe. Put everything in writing and have it reviewed by an attorney no matter how trivial or trite it may seem. Heavy-duty legalese documents are especially necessary for associates. Put these guys through the Trials of Job or the Labors of Hercules before even considering bringing them on as partners.

    Whoever said the basis for all human relations is trust obviously was some sort of gullible dimwit who never had to deal with the people you know. You have come to understand all too well how people envy you for your success, your money, and your extraordinary talent which is why you need to be on guard twenty-four seven. The minute you start trusting is the minute people start getting too close and you get hurt. Once they draw blood, these piranhas will make a skeletal carcass out of you in a heartbeat. So keep your people at arm's length, don't open up, and always keep up the "holier than thou" doctor persona wall at all costs.

As a general rule, when trust is the issue, consider the past. Look at how many times you've been burned before. Haven't you learned your lesson yet? The only one you can truly trust is you. Your best bet is a safe and secure personal hell of seclusion, isolation, aversion and paranoia to protect yourself and your precious practice from harm. Besides, you're a one-man show anyway, surrounded by a bunch of lurking vultures waiting for signs of weakness.

Therefore, hire family and friends to fill out the ranks just like your very own Republican Guard. Hey, they may not know much about dentistry, but they're a lot less likely to turn on you especially when it comes to all the unethical stuff you pull on your patients. Since you have their ignorance and undying loyalty, you will be well insulated from any attacks that are bound to come your way.

"It's a well-known practice development fact that you're never going to make any money trying to build your practice from the inside out with the warm trusting relationships that already exist right under your nose."

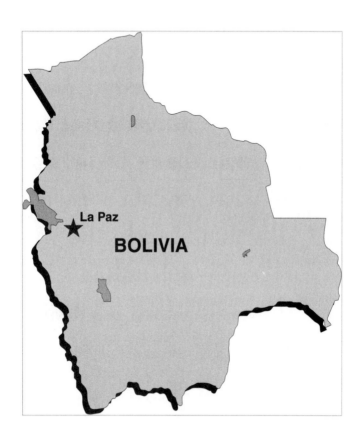

15

Pump All of Your Money Into Marketing

The main problem with you is, you just don't get it! The $25,000 a month yellow pages ad with the pullout centerfold of you and your 68 smiling staff members is not going to cut it. The full-color glossy portfolios with the eight staggered laminated sheets, and the CD-rom business card you mail to the 21,337 homes in your zip code every month at the cost of the gross national product of Bolivia are totally insufficient. The interactive practice newsletter complete with its racy jokes, off-color humor, and downloadable e-coupons for "buy one get one free" cleanings is nothing but a drop in the bucket. Therefore, you need to get serious about ratcheting up your marketing.

It's a well-known practice development fact that you're never going to make any money trying to build your practice from the inside out with the warm trusting relationships that already exist right under your nose. You know too damn well that all the incomplete and not accepted treatment these people have piled up over the years has been a tremendous waste of your time. What you need is fresh meat and lots of it. The new people obviously will trust you more, need less education, and will blindly do whatever you tell them to do without question, because anyone ingenious enough to hire the Goodyear Blimp to circle the city all day with their face on the Jumbotron, has *got* to be good. Besides, you need to keep the new patient carousel going, as in, "in one door and out the other." You have to figure, with your 90% attrition rate, even at 200 new patients a month, you're struggling. Remember there's lots of dummies out there who have not caught on to the dentistry fad and simply do not appreciate the beauty of sky-writing.

Therefore, at least half of your overhead should be marketing. It's already at 75% you say? Excellent! But whatever you do, never ever keep statistics or tabs on your return on investment such as how effective your marketing is at bringing in quality patients that are right for your practice, or if the marketing is bringing in anybody at all for that matter. Just keep haphazardly pouring money into every dental promotional and marketing gimmick known to mankind and you're bound to hit on something that works sooner or later – usually later, much later, like after you're flat, busted broke. Which is, of course, what you're shooting for here aren't you?

"It cannot be stressed enough that most people have no lives anyway, especially in comparison to your 'Lifestyles of the Rich and Famous' standards."

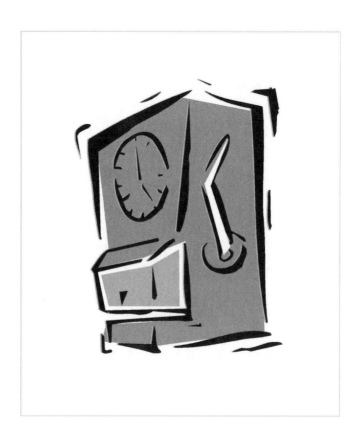

16

Never Be on Time

Never, ever wear a watch. Believe that time is just an abstract concept. On time is when you get there. Start late. Run over. This is your executive privilege. Having the honor of coming to your practice is the highlight of your patient's day. It cannot be stressed enough that most people have no lives anyway, especially in comparison to your "Lifestyles of the Rich and Famous" standards. Their world revolves around your hand piece. Being on time is overrated. The early bird gets the worm is a flawed theory (ever tried waiting in line all night for Springsteen tickets? – it guarantees you squat). Learn a lesson from your appointment book: These people have been booked months in advance, and do they show up on time if at all? Of course not. Also be sure to have a "keep them waiting next time" patient list to really fix their wagons. When they do decide to show up again and grace you with their presence, you'll know what to do.

Now, as for staff being on time, this is a whole different ball of wax. When staff is late, time is money. When you are late, time is being wisely spent handling the pool builder, Porsche dealer, your stock broker, or your bookie, to name a few. By the way, there's no better time to talk to your spouse than when you have a patient in the chair—as in "Hi spouse, it's me...yeah she's numbing up so it'll be awhile. So tell me about your entire day from the moment you woke-up until now..."that sort of thing. Be sure to institute the: "59 policy" (in a minute early out a minute early) to ensure maximum productivity and no risk of any overtime. Do the math and you'll find that over the course of a year this adds up to over one one-hundredth of a monthly payment for the new Hummer you so richly deserve.

The other aspect of time that's probably driving you nuts is hygiene. Those incessant buzzers, lights, and bells going off and all those requests for exams, checks and consults...and for what? So a patient comes back for another lousy $80 prophy? Puhlease...it makes you wonder why you bother having a hygiene department at all. Not only would you save all that wasted time running around like a dentist with his head cut off, but think of the money you'll save by not having to pay $30-$40k per hygienist! Restorative and cosmetics are where the bucks are, and you really never need to be on time with these people because they understand that the precision artistry and quality of your work is measured by how long it takes you to get the job done. An hour and a half for a filling? Now there's value being created.

Finally, to avoid any misunderstandings, make sure that your staff has a clear understanding about ending the day on time. As they say in New Jersey, "Fuggedda 'bout it"! You do some of your best work at night and often on patients. If you've got a chance to pull in an extra $950 for doing some work in another quad, go for it. Dispense with the senseless formalities of patient and staff agreement. Drill first and ask questions later.

Not keeping your word is an effective practice management tool to provide an insecure and uncertain environment to keep people just confused enough for you to maintain control.

17

Don't Keep Your Word about Anything

Walk your talk? The tongue in your shoe should match the tongue in your mouth? These are the ridiculous ideals of Utopian pop psychology. So lose the Dr. Phil complex, and get down to the brass tacks of how to truly have more freedom, fulfillment, and financial gain in practice. Do exactly what you want, when you want, and how you want it to the exclusion of everyone else. The best office policies are the ones that you come up with off the top of your head and verbally announce to your team as law, and the ones you already have agreement on that you feel like changing on the fly because they suddenly don't work for you anymore. When you are struck by genius, by all means stop what you are doing and get your people on your new project or idea ASAP right in the middle of the day. This should also contribute quite nicely to creating a chaotic working environment (see next chapter). Keeping your word doesn't keep your staff on their toes. Breaking promises, finding loopholes, and being changeable without apparent rhyme or reason, will definitely keep your patients and staff from feeling too secure and confident. You sure as hell don't want them getting the crazy notion that they have the upper hand, which as you know has a tendency to lead to a revolt of the masses. You don't want to end up with the Smile Center of Stalingrad, do you? Not keeping your word is an effective practice management tool to provide an insecure and uncertain environment to keep people just confused enough for you to maintain control. This technique is also useful in hiring new people.

The secret to snagging good personnel is to promise them the moon, lead them down the primrose path, and once you've lured them into your web, pull the old black widow spider maneuver. They're not going anywhere. They are leveraged by their family and their bills. Start slowly with having them cover some nights. Then Saturdays, just for the 300-day probationary period. Later they can go back to 9-3 with an hour lunch that they said you originally promised. When the probationary period is up, make sure you forget their date of hire, misplace their personnel file (if you even have one), and keep putting off any request for a review until they give up.

Keeping your word with patients doesn't benefit you either. Suppose you lay out a treatment plan they can accept and agree to, but once you get started, voila! Lo and behold, wouldn't you know it, there's all this additional add-on work to be done. You don't want to be locked into some rigid agreement. That kind of thing always ends up hitting you in the wallet. So when the work is done and six fillings have become six crowns, let them argue about the $5,000 difference with the front desk. Besides, this strategy is a lot less risky than putting that kind of money in the market. Even if you don't collect, you have your lawyers and personal Gestapo agents working the finance department to straighten things out. Now isn't this a blissful way of building trust and credibility?

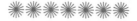

"People coming into a serene and organized office that is neat, clean, and smoothly run generally freaks them out and makes them suspicious of your ulterior motives such as expecting a lot of money for your treatment to pay for all your snappy Feng Shui décor."

18

Create a Chaotic Work Environment

Chaos creates cash! The more frantic and stressful the practice operates, the more successful it appears to others. People coming into a serene and organized office that is neat, clean, and smoothly run generally freaks them out and makes them suspicious of your ulterior motives, such as expecting a lot of money for your treatment to pay for all your snappy Feng Shui décor. Like attracts like, and since 90% of patients come in with some degree of anxiety and stress, they should feel right at home in the three-ring circus you've got going. If you're having trouble visualizing how the office environment should be, just picture the floor of the Stock Exchange. The frenetic pace, money changing hands like mad…you've got the idea. Steer clear of the spa-like setting fad that's been sweeping across the field of dentistry like a plague of locusts. Candles, new age music, massage, aromatherapy, and tropical fish – it's all enough to put someone to sleep. Then how ya' gonna charge them for gas? You didn't consider that little consequence did you, Dr. Doolittle? Save the fluff for the fruitcakes who run the Spiritual Enlightenment and Wellness of Being Resort down the street. There's no money in pampering people with impeccable service and loving attention.

So the lesson here is keep your people busy, nonstop all the time. Lord knows you're paying them enough. Pile on the projects, send them off on tangents (i.e. your next multi-level marketing scheme), and be sure to give them plenty of your extraneous personal extras to do in their spare time, such as booking your next cruise and ordering your new clubs. And why hire a dedicated recare coordinator when the hygienist you have is just sitting around bored to tears? Get her on the phone to track down non-compliant patients. If she gets pissed off at you for forcing her to do this, don't worry. Her annoyed and aggravated tone is just what your patients need to motivate them to come in. The guiltier you can make the patient, the better, so when they arrive they'll just add to the Mardi Gras–like atmosphere.

Some other noteworthy essentials include heaps of clutter, loud machines with exposed wiring, and half-eaten food and drinks piled behind a small, sliding glass window at the front desk. You many want to consider opening a Dairy Queen out there for everyone's convenience, particularly your patients since they're going to be there awhile anyway. And on the subject of the front desk, you must institute a surefire way to cover yourself and guard against broken and cancelled appointments while keeping the place hopping. Play the odds and triple book *everything*, especially recall appointments. Push lab-ins and suture removals off until later or move them to another day. No rush there. You've already got their money.

The most effective way to create chaos is to make sure everyone is cross-trained and doing each other's job. For example, don't separate duties and responsibilities at the front desk so that one person is accountable for financial arrangements and another is handling the schedule. Just have everyone maintain an "all hands on deck" mentality and have them grab whatever comes their way at any time. This is how you get things done fast and furiously.

Finally, just to keep things interesting (and give yourself a break) call your office just before the start of a day, and have them cancel out your schedule at the last possible minute. This will allow you to discover just how ingenious and efficient your people really are while allowing you to make your tee time. Fore!

※※※※※※

"A stallion's gotta roam my friend, and the entrepreneurial spirit cannot be bridled in you."

19

Work First, Family Second

That's right. Everyone in the family wants to live in the lap of luxury, with the 126" plasma T.V.; the 3,000 square foot heated in-ground pool with the waterfall and hot tub; the five car garage for the two Beemers, the Jag, the Navigator, and the Ferrari for tooling around on the weekends; the Armani suits…wait, that's all for you. Well they all want the expensive toys, too. Yet it never ceases to amaze how they whine and complain about how you're never home, how they never see you anymore, how you're missing their formative years, and how you're having an affair with Ms. Hottie Hygienist. It gets a bit old after a while, doesn't it? All you're out doing every day (besides the hygienist) is raking in piles of money and being a good provider – Is that so wrong? Of course not, you've got your priorities straight. A stallion's gotta roam my friend, and the entrepreneurial spirit cannot be bridled in you. You have a vision that cannot become clouded by birthdays, anniversaries, school functions, vacations, and Christmas. You have been called to the profession in much the same way a man is called to the priesthood, except you get paid obscene amounts of money and can skip mass on Sunday to be in the office.

Without you in the office there would be anarchy — well, at least more anarchy than usual. Production would go to Hell in a handbasket in two days flat. And your staff would be completely lost and purposeless without your commanding presence guiding them through the stormy seas of dentistry. Meanwhile, back at the ranch (or the 15 bedroom, 11 bath Georgian Manor home if you prefer), you're buried in years of back projects the wife's been saving up for you. Then there's these strange, little aliens called "children" who keep tormenting you for attention. At least at the office you get paid for this type of torture, or could cut someone loose if need be. Can't do that at home without it costing you a bundle, so you're better off at work.

So to summarize, a woman's place is in the home, children should be seen but not heard, and you put in an 80-hour work week and yet another big fat nail into the coffin of your demise. Congratulations!

"Start off by loading him up with all the kids and extractions you can pack into a day while making sure he's got all your nights and weekends covered."

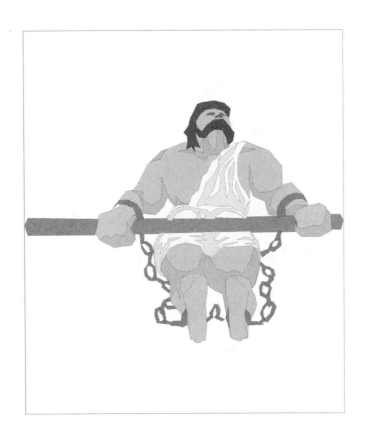

20

Hire a Slave Not an Associate

Do you remember in Conan the Barbarian when they abducted Arnold as a young boy after murdering his family, and enslaved him for roughly 20 years of daily back-breaking labor until he finally earned his freedom by winning fame and fortune for his master in the gladiator pits? That's exactly what you need to do when looking to hire an associate. It's recommended, however, that you skip murdering the guy's family and giving him a sword if at all possible, but other than that…A bit severe you say? Look, that's the only thing these Gen X'ers and Gen Y'ers coming out of dental school these days understand. All of them have the work ethic of a three-toed sloth (with all apologies to the species), and are just as motivated to earn the quarter mill they want to make right out of the box. Hell, you'd like to make that kind of money yourself! They gotta suffer to succeed just like you did. You haven't been in practice 10 years just to pay some hot shot Eddie Vedder look-a-like's student loan back in his first six months of practice. To further emphasize your point, you may want to flip the guy a copy of The Seven Habits of Highly Successful People to read and ask him if it rings any bells. If not, hire him on the spot. This is just the type of unambitious sucker you're looking for.

Start off by loading him up with all the kids and extractions you can pack into a day while making sure he's got all your nights and weekends covered. Then put him in the hole – a.k.a. the 70's throwback room with the brown paneling, vomit yellow chair, lava lamp, and the pooka beads for a door. Finally make sure he gets all the used instruments, your old hand piece, and the one-armed assistant with bad b.o. and cataracts. Oh, and on his day off, make sure you have him out doing magic tricks and giving out brochures at the local nursery school to drum up some new business.

When in doubt, simply download all of your scut work onto this guy until he's put in his mandatory 20 years to life and is ready to enter into his indentured servitude agreement – in other words, a partnership.

"There's nothing that says revenge like a nice hefty lawsuit or legal action taken against anyone who would dare owe you $100 or more."

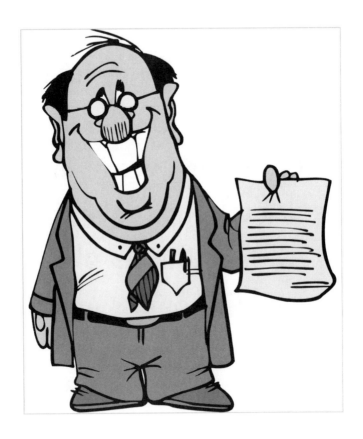

21

Keep a Lawyer In Your Back Pocket

You think you have it bad? After dentists, lawyers are the last professionals to be paid for their services. On the hierarchical totem pole of who the universe screws over the most, there is actually someone out there worse off than you. So here's how you both win: Retain a lawyer, keep him on call, and let "sue, sue, sue before they do" become your motto. As a matter of fact, make sure you have reams of your lawyer's letterhead on hand (just in case) and work, "you'll be hearing from my lawyers", into your daily vocabulary.

There's nothing that says revenge like a nice hefty lawsuit or legal action taken against anyone who would dare owe you $100 or more. Never mind that legal fees can run you thousands of dollars- it's well worth it. First, because nothing puts the fear of God into your patients and vendors like a subpoena, and secondly because you're probably not going to pay the attorney fees like everyone else anyway. Be sure, however, not to let the poor bastard know that until you've cracked at least the six-figure mark in legal services. Don't worry, he's used to getting shafted just like you, and he has a pretty thick skin for unethical behavior. "Birds of a feather...", remember?

In America you are only innocent until you run out of money, so be sure and go after as many people as you can who cannot afford to defend themselves for any length of time. Just remember, legal battles are time consuming, so have your appointment coordinator block out time in your daily production schedule to be available for all those counsel calls, depositions, and court appearances-all of which, by the way, are a real hoot and very empowering. Before you know it, you'll be reaping the rewards from small claims court settlements and car repossessions. So, there you have it – another great source of residual income and another feather in your cap for your many contributions for the good of humanity.

"You know how you've been considering calling in an interior decorator and a contractor to remodel and renovate a facility that has all the modern charm of a 19th century log cabin?"

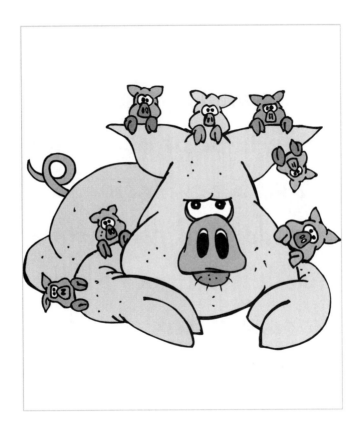

22

Keep Your Facility Like a Pig Sty

You know how you've been feeling a bit depressed lately because your office has begun to take on the look and feel of your college dorm room? You know all those thoughts you've been having about renting a 50 yard dumpster to haul away all the garbage that's been piling up for the last 15 years? You know how you've been considering calling in an interior decorator and a contractor to remodel and renovate a facility that has all the modern charm of a 19th century log cabin? You know how you've just about had it with the mice, cockroaches, and the squirrel nesting in the autoclave? And you know how you made a New Year's resolution to change all that? Well, you better knock off that forward thinking faster than you can say linoleum. Why risk losing possible government funding for the little landfill project you've been putting so much time into developing all these years? Hey, if the junk gets a little deeper you might even qualify for "Ripley's Believe It or Not". Now there's a tourist attraction for ya'. Imagine lines of tour buses filled with site seers hoping to catch a glimpse of the World's Most Horrific Dental Practice. Just think of the new patient opportunities!

The tour could begin with a little stroll down Marlboro Way (the walkway up to the front door), where people can try to sidestep the lipstick coated cigarette butts and matted medallions of Bubble Yum. Next up, the reception area, replete with cobweb-laden silk flower arrangements, moss covered fish tank, strewn kids toys, and yellowing magazines. Strolling along the frayed and stained indoor/outdoor carpet to the front desk area, tourists can marvel at the mysterious frosted sliding doors wondering what lies hidden beyond. Perhaps the myriad of multicolored stickers and plaques plastered about this portal would give some inkling...MC, VISA, AMEX, Rotary, NRA, "Miss an appointment and I breaka you face" bumper sticker...It's up to them to decide what it all means. The tour would weave it's way from here down an obstacle course of boxes and crates to the rooms where the Medieval barber works (that's you by the way). Here people can see all the tools and instruments of the trade, both before and after use, laid out in their blood encrusted glory basking in the dim illumination of your overhead insect collection display cases (that's right, the light fixtures). They can even feed the squirrel as they leave. So it's probably a good idea to have one of those pellet-filled gumball machines on hand.

If you charge about five bucks a head, half-price for children, plus the new patients and rodent residuals, you're looking at some serious simoleons at the end of the month. What about OSHA you ask? OSHA, schmosha, since when has that ever stopped you? Besides, you've got a lawyer, remember?

"A truly great person such as yourself is to be envied and revered despite your malicious, unethical, and self-centered way of life."

23

Make a Lot of Enemies

Burn bridges. Hold grudges. Be rancorous. Rankle everyone you come into contact with, and there you have it.

There's not a quicker way to do yourself and your practice in than surrounding yourself with people who would like nothing more than to see you rot in the fiery pits of Hell as you suffer all eternity undergoing infinite root canal (and no, there isn't any Novocain in Hell). Napoleon was right when he said you can measure how great you are by the number of enemies you have, and he pretty much ruled the whole damn world at one time in history, didn't he?

A truly great person such as yourself is to be envied and revered despite your malicious, unethical, and self-centered way of life. Remember that people dislike or hate you because they are jealous of you and your wealth, power, and influence, not as a consequence of treating other human beings with disrespect, disinterest, and a complete lack of empathy.

Your goal is to change the world to suit your own ends, and dentistry is the vehicle you have chosen to crush your adversaries beneath the juggernaut of your needs, wants, and desires. There's nothing wrong with a touch of megalomania tempered with just the right amount of manipulation and deceit which eventually makes for some thoroughly vengeful enemies out there looking to ruin you at any time.

Now if all of this sounds so wildly pathetic as to be insane, you really do have some work to do. Otherwise, given the path you are on it is recommended you practice your Shakespeare, as in "Et tu, Brute?"

"Whoever gave you the insane idea that paying for quality pays off, never saw your lab and supply bills."

24

Cut Corners

So how do you really lower your overhead and save a small fortune in the process? That's right, by cutting corners every chance you get. Whoever gave you the insane idea that paying for quality pays off, never saw your lab and supply bills. Truth is, this is just the sort of thing that eats into profits and keeps you up nights giving you worry wrinkles. Face it, a trained monkey with some Plaster of Paris and a jar of paste could handle your lab work just as well as those rip-off artists you're dealing with now. Patients will never know the difference-unless you forget to tell them to only eat soft foods and drink through a straw for the rest of their lives. Oh yeah, and tell them never to smile again either – very important. Then there's the matter of supplies and equipment. So have pencil and paper handy and take down these gems.

The following is a short list of commonly used yet unnecessary or wasteful equipment and supplies with their much cheaper, more utile alternatives:

Dumb

Composite
bonding material

Cotton rolls

Latex gloves

X-ray film

Curing light

High speed drill

Smart

Quick-Crete
(and it lasts and lasts).

Polyester or rayon rolls
(they breathe better).

Gardening gloves
(they're absorbent,
washable, and reusable).

Polaroid film (no more waiting, no more patient fear, saves on costly developing and chemicals).

Blow-torch (bonds in two seconds and your patients will think twice about ever getting another cavity; ensures recare).

Hammer and chisel (a bit barbaric, but people expect this from a dentist: hammer also saves on anesthesia).

Autoclave	Microwave (a few more sparks, but try doing your Cup O' Noodles simultaneously in an autoclave-it ain't happening)
Ultrasonic Sterilizer	"As Seen on T.V." sonic jewelry cleaner (must there be an explanation, duh?)

Now as far as time saving techniques go, start with hygiene. Ditch the scaling and cavitron, and get right to the nitty gritty. It's all about looking good, and what your patients can't see, can't hurt them. They're there for the pearly whites so polish 'em up good and send them on their merry way. Think of how much your productivity just jumped with this beauty. Yes, they'll be back in time, but for the good stuff like full mouth restorations with implants. And remember to do your part by performing quick and shoddy, half-assed dentistry so that their crowns (along with the remainder of their dental health) fail within the first couple of years.

Lastly, rid yourself of the financial burden of all those valueless extra staff. This basically equates to anyone not producing at least $40,000 in closed cases a month. The rest are just riding the coattails of your success. And you were wondering why your back hurts.

"What you really need is to slow everything down to a nice torpid pace by being chemically disconnected from your nervous system."

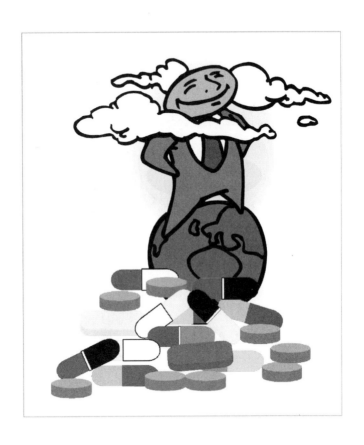

25

Start the Day with a Large Dose of Anti-Depressants

Okay, listen up and listen good. You're almost there and this one should put you over the top. Here's the number one way to destroy your practice and, as an added bonus, the rest of your life as well! All you have to do is wake up in the morning, groggily stumble to the medicine cabinet (which is no doubt filled with the other 10-15 drugs that you are on), and pop a few Prozac, Paxil, Zoloft, or whatever floats your boat, and magically the whole world quickly becomes wonderful place just like that!

You know all those horrible ideas and thoughts that you've been having about fear, failure, and rejection? Just replace those with happy thoughts brought on by a drug-induced stupor. Not only will this handle the true cause of those negative feelings, once and for all, it will also handle all those hundreds of other feelings you've been having that take up so much of your time like joy, enthusiasm, exhilaration, and sexual arousal – yikes, that's a bore for you.

What you really need is to slow everything down to a nice torpid pace by being chemically disconnected from your nervous system which, by the way, is probably one of those excess organs the medical and psychiatric professions say people suffer from anyway- kind of like your appendix, your tonsils, and the pre-frontal lobe of your brain. Who needs 'em? Not you, that's for sure, because anti-depressants are the silver bullet to all of what ills the mind and body.

What about spirituality you ask? It's a bunch of new age crapola. Man is nothing but a stimulus response animal - a hunk of biologically animated meat worth about $1.98 in chemicals (a couple hundred dollars more if you've got enough of the good stuff coursing through your veins when you finally kick the bucket). The drug companies and the psych's know what they're doing, so you're in good hands. It's done wonders for Tony Soprano, and it works even better for you because you're not in organized crime, you're a dentist. Only those weak-willed, bad guy types who go on Prozac have manic, suicidal, and homicidal tendencies, not a respectable, professional person such as you. Plus, you are aiding your fellow man when you take these types of drugs. What do you think would happen if you stopped taking Prozac and, as a result, people found out that they could get mentally and physically well without drugs? Why it would be total insanity caused by the collapse of the multi-billion dollar pharmaceutical industry that exists solely for the well being of mankind. All because you had to run off half-cocked, find spirituality, and tap into the unlimited power of the mind. So don't get any bright ideas that will take you off the straight and narrow.

The Dalai Lama? He's a clown. Deepak Chopra? An idiot. Tony Robbins. A kook. Buddha? Mad. Stick with reliable, modern science and go with the quick fix route to sanity, mental health, and personal fulfillment. It's for a good cause after all. So show your allegiance by taking anti-depressants, and maybe even naming your dogs after a couple of the more popular brands.

Afterward

Congratulations! You made it. If you've been reading carefully and taking notes, you should soon be well on your way to becoming one of those "four out of five dentists surveyed of their patients who chew gum" – because participation in a farcical sugarless gum poll is about all you'll have left going for you once you've seriously applied what's in this book. Now in reading this book if you found yourself unamused and intensely interested in getting down to the business of making some changes to better model yourself and your practice after as many chapters as possible, that's just perfect. You've seen the light, or in this case, the darkness. However, if you found yourself laughing or shaking your head with dropped-jawed astonishment as you read this material, you really missed the boat. We're sorry to say that you're probably going to have to settle for a successful practice and a fulfilling life. Knowing your type, you'll most likely become even more fixated on bettering yourself to pompously avoid becoming or doing anything that is remotely related to what you've just read. Suit yourself. You get what you deserve.

But as for the now truly edified of you who have taken this book to heart, hopefully you've discovered the secret message outlined herein: the universe does in fact completely revolve around you, the God of Dentistry. No rules or laws of any sort apply to you. The true path to enlightenment and success lies down the road of self-absorption, know-it-allness, and selfishness. People can advise and perhaps urge you otherwise until the cows come home, but you know better. This book speaks to the core of who you are and how the practice of dentistry in its ideal state should be.

You've got the big picture now – and God help us all.

American Dental Association
Dept. of Library Services